NUTRITIONAL TREATMENT FOR GOITRE DISEASE.

By

DR DOUGLAS JASON

TABLE OF CONTENTS

ABOUT THE AUTHOR

INTRODUCTION

TABLE OF CONTENTS

NUTRITIONAL TREATMENT FOR GOITRE DISEASE.

INTRODUCTION

Part 1:UNDERSTANDING GOITER.

Part 2: Wholesome Establishments Keeping up with Thyroid Wellbeing.

Part 3: IODINE; THE Urgent Component.

Part 4: SELENIUM AND THYROID Capability.

Part 5: Offsetting THYROID Chemicals WITH Supplements.

Part 6: DIETARY Procedures FOR GOITER The board.

Part 7: Way of life CHANGES FOR GOITER Avoidance.

Part 8. Key Dietary Methodologies:

CONCLUSION

ABOUT THE AUTHOR

Dr. DOUGLAS JASON is a certified dietician who has a strong passion for wellness and a big eagerness to help people all over the world. He uses healthy food, herbs, sauce, and other useful tools to help mankind realize its overall goal of optimum health.

INTRODUCTION

Overseeing goitre sicknesses includes an exhaustive methodology pointed toward tending to the extension of the thyroid organ. Goiter, frequently brought about by iodine inadequacy or other thyroid problems, requires cautious thought of both clinical and way-of-life intercessions. This presentation will dig into the different features of overseeing goitre, including demonstrative methods, treatment choices, and the significance of keeping a sound thyroid capability for general prosperity.

Part 1:UNDERSTANDING GOITER.

<u>Definition and Kinds of Goiter</u>:
A goitre is an expansion or development of the thyroid organ, which is situated at the foundation of the neck. This condition is frequently noticeable and can go in size from a little knob to an enormous mass. There are a few kinds of goitre, characterizes view of their causes and qualities.
<u>Straightforward or Colloid</u>
<u>Goiter:</u> This is the most widely recognized type, frequently

brought about by iodine lack, prompting the thyroid's endeavour to repay by amplifying.

Endemic Goiter: Connected to explicit geological locales with low iodine levels in the dirt and water, bringing about a higher pervasiveness of goitre in those areas.

Harmful Goiter (Graves' Illness): This type includes an immune system reaction, where the resistant framework erroneously goes after the thyroid organ, prompting its expansion and overproduction of thyroid chemicals.

Multinodular Goiter: Described by the improvement of different knobs in the thyroid organ, making it extend. This might be located with iodine inadequacy or different elements.

Reasons for Goiter:

Understanding the reasons for goitre is urgent for compelling administration and counteraction.

Iodine Inadequacy: An absence of iodine in the eating routine is an essential driver, as iodine is fundamental for the creation of thyroid chemicals.

Immune system Infections:

Conditions like Graves' illness can make the safe framework assault the thyroid, prompting goitre.

Thyroiditis: Aggravation of the thyroid, frequently because of contaminations or immune system problems, can add to goitre improvement.

Hereditary Variables: A few people might be hereditarily inclined toward foster goitre, particularly on the off chance that there is a family background of thyroid problems.

Side effects of Goiter:

The side effects of goitre are given its size and fundamental reason.

Apparent Expanding: Development of the thyroid organ is many times observable as an enlarging at the foundation of the neck.

<u>Trouble Gulping or Relaxing:</u>
Enormous goitres might apply tension on the throat or windpipe, prompting trouble in gulping or relaxing.

<u>Roughness:</u> Tension on the vocal lines because of a developed thyroid can bring about a raspy voice.

<u>Thyroid Brokenness:</u> Contingent upon the sort of goitre, people might encounter side effects of hyperthyroidism (unreasonable thyroid chemical creation) or hypothyroidism (lacking thyroid chemical creation).

<u>Contextual analyses:</u>
Iodine Lack in Nepal: A review directed in districts of Nepal

uncovered a high occurrence of basic goitre because of iodine lack. Carrying out iodized salt projects fundamentally decreased the predominance of goitre here. Graves' Sickness and Thyroid **Expansion:** A case report featured the association between Graves' infection and thyroid development, underlining the requirement for early finding and suitable administration to forestall entanglements.

Down to earth Tips:
Guarantee Sufficient Iodine Admission: Devouring iodized salt or food rich in iodine, like fish, can assist with forestalliodlack-related goitre.

<u>Standard Thyroid Check-ups:</u>

People with a family background of thyroid issues or living in iodine-lacking districts ought to go through normal thyroid capability tests. ounscounseledical services Prolfvent that you notice side effects of goitre, for example, expanding, trouble gulping, or voice changes, look for clinical guidance immediately for an exhaustive assessment. Understanding goitre includes perceiving its sorts, knowing the causes, monitoring side effects, and executing reasonable measures for avoidance and the executives.

Part 2: Wholesome Establishments Keeping up with Thyroid Wellbeing.

This chapter delves into the basic job that fundamental supplements play in saving ideal thyroid capability. The understanding-boggling connection between sustenance and thyroid wellbeing is vital for people looking to upgrade their general prosperity.

1. Significance of Fundamental Supplements:

The thyroid, a little butterfly-molded organ in the neck, is a force to be reckoned with for controlling digestion, energy creation, and in general hormonal equilibrium. Fundamental supplements, including nutrients and minerals, act as the structure blocks for thyroid chemicals. These chemicals, specifically thyroxine (T4) and triiodothyronine (T3) are critical for different physiological cycles.

2. Job of Iodine:

Iodine stands apart as a foundation of thyroid wellbeing. It is a critical part of thyroid chemicals, and a lack can prompt circumstances like goitre and hypothyroidism. Contextual analyses have shown populaces with inadequate iodine consumption experience higher paces of thyroid problems. **Reasonable tip:** Consolidate iodine-rich food varieties like ocean growth, iodized salt, and fish into your eating regimen to guarantee a sufficient inventory.

3. Selenium's Critical Job:

The fact that influences thyroid capability makes selenium another fundamental mineral. It is an indispensable piece of chemicals liable for changing T4 over completely to the more dynamic T3 chemical. Selenium lack has been connected to an expanded gamble of thyroid infections. Functional tip: Incorporate selenium-rich food sources, for example, Brazil nuts, sunflower seeds, and fish to help ideal thyroid movement.

4. **Key Minerals Past Iodine and Selenium:**

Aside from iodine and selenium, different minerals assume essential parts of thyroid well-being. Zinc, for example, is fundamental for the blend of thyroid chemicals, while iron is urgent for their legitimate digestion. Remembering various supplement-thick food sources for your eating routine guarantees an exhaustive stockpile of these minerals.

5. **Contextual analyses:**

A few examinations have researched the effect of

nourishment on thyroid wellbeing. For example, a review led in locales with iodine-lacking soils exhibited a critical decrease in thyroid problems following iodine supplementation programs. Essentially, research has featured the positive relationship between selenium consumption and a lower rate of immune system thyroid circumstances.

6. Functional Tips for Ideal Thyroid Nourishment:

a. Differentiate Your Eating regimen: Consume a shifted diet rich in organic products, vegetables, entire grains, lean proteins, and dairy.

b. Screen Iodine Admission: Be aware of iodine levels, particularly assuming that you live in regions with low iodine in the dirt.

c. Consider Selenium Enhancements: In conference with medical care proficient, consider selenium supplements on the off chance that your eating routine needs adequate selenium-rich food varieties.

d. Balance Micronutrients: Guarantee a satisfactory admission of zinc, iron, and different minerals through an even eating regimen.

the crucial job of fundamental supplements in keeping up with ideal thyroid well-being. By

grasping the significance of
iodine, selenium, and other key
minerals, people can settle on
informed dietary decisions to help
a sound and working thyroid
organ.

Part 3: IODINE; THE Urgent Component.

Iodine assumes an urgent part in keeping up with ideal well-being, especially in forestalling and treating goitre, a condition described by the growth of the thyroid organ. This part investigates the diverse meanings of iodine, digging into its natural capabilities, the pervasiveness of goitre, and reasonable methodologies for guaranteeing sufficient iodine consumption.

Iodine and Goiter: A More Profound Association

Goiter, basically brought about by iodine lack, highlights the basic job iodine plays in thyroid capability. The thyroid organ, a butterfly-molded organ in the neck, depends on iodine to create thyroid chemicals thyroxine (T4) and triiodothyronine (T3). At the point when iodine levels are lacking, the thyroid augments trying to catch additional iodine from the circulation system, prompting goitre.

To outline this association, consider the contextual analysis of a local area in a district with generally low iodine levels in the dirt. Through far-reaching iodine supplementation drives, specialists noticed a huge decrease in goitre pervasiveness more than quite a while. This case features the immediate relationship between iodine accessibility and goitre occurrence, underlining the significance of iodine in thyroid well-being.

Iodine-Rich Food varieties:
Building a Fair Eating regimen
An essential part of keeping up with sufficient iodine levels is integrating iodine-rich food varieties into one's eating regimen. Fish, like fish and ocean growth, is an eminent wellspring of iodine. Contextual analyses led in populaces with maximum usage of fish uncover lower frequencies of iodine lack issues, exhibiting

the positive effect of dietary decisions on thyroid wellbeing. Furthermore, dairy items, eggs, and certain products of the soil add to iodine admission. The part gives a far-reaching rundown of iodine-rich food varieties, permitting perusers to settle on informed dietary decisions to help thyroid capability.

Supplementation Procedures: Exploring Choices
In districts where iodine-rich food sources are scant or dietary inclinations limit iodine consumption, supplementation turns into a reasonable arrangement. The section investigates different iodine

supplementation choices, including iodized salt, iodine supplements, and sustained food sources. It digs into the viability of these systems and offers useful ways to integrate them into everyday schedules.

Drawing on research discoveries, the part underlines the significance of balance in iodine supplementation, as extreme admission can likewise prompt unfavourable well-being impacts. It gives rules for deciding individual iodine needs founded on elements like age, orientation, and well-being status.

Enabling Wellbeing Through Iodine Mindfulness

enlightening the critical job of iodine in forestalling and treating goitre. Through a mix of logical bits of knowledge, contextual investigations, and commonsense tips, perusers gain a far-reaching comprehension of the significant meaning of iodine in thyroid well-being. Equipped with this information, people can settle on informed choices to guarantee ideal iodine consumption and advance by and large prosperity.

Part 4: SELENIUM AND THYROID Capability.

Selenium, a fundamental minor component, assumes a critical part in keeping up with ideal thyroid capability. This part investigates the complex connection between selenium lack and goitre, revealing insight into the significance of this mineral in thyroid well-being.

1. Selenium Inadequacy and Goiter:

Selenium inadequacy has been firmly connected to the improvement of goitre, a condition described by the extension of the thyroid organ. The thyroid organ depends on selenium for the creation of selenoproteins, especially selenoprotein N and thyroxine deiodinase. These proteins are fundamental for the combination and guideline of thyroid chemicals.

Contextual investigations: Various examinations have recorded the commonness of goitre in locales with selenium-lacking soils. For example, a review led in specific areas of China, where selenium levels in the dirt are low, uncovered a higher occurrence of goitre among the populace.

Pragmatic Tips:

a. Customary selenium testing:
People in districts with low selenium levels ought to think about standard testing to screen their selenium status.

b. Dietary broadening:
Remembering selenium-rich food sources for the eating routine, for example, Brazil nuts, fish, and poultry, can assist with forestalling lack.

<u>2. Selenium-rich food varieties</u>:
Understanding selenium-rich food varieties is vital for keeping up with sufficient levels of this minor component. Integrating these food sources into one's eating regimen can add to general thyroid well-being.

Key Food varieties:

a. Brazil Nuts: Among the most extravagant wellsprings of selenium, consuming only a couple of nuts can meet the day-to-day selenium prerequisite.

b. Fish: Fish, shellfish, and scavengers are brilliant wellsprings of selenium.

c. Poultry: Chicken and turkey are dependable wellsprings of selenium.

d. Entire Grains: Earthy coloured rice, oats, and entire wheat bread contain selenium, adding to a reasonable eating regimen.

3. Advantages of Supplementation:

While getting selenium from a balanced eating routine is great, supplementation can be gainful for people in danger of lack or those with explicit ailments.

Contemplations:

a. Thyroid Problems: People with thyroid issues, particularly those influencing selenium digestion, may profit from designated supplementation.

b. Geological Variables: Inhabitants of areas with selenium-inadequate soils might require enhancements to meet their dietary necessities.

Selenium is a basic component for thyroid well-being, and its inadequacy is firmly connected with the improvement of goitre. By understanding the significance of selenium-rich food sources and taking into account supplementation when important, people can find proactive ways to help their thyroid capability and by and large prosperity.

Part 5: Offsetting THYROID Chemicals WITH Supplements.

We are investigating the unpredictable connection between fundamental supplements and thyroid capability, zeroing in on the effect of key nutrients and omega-3 unsaturated fats. Nutrients A, D, and B:

Vitamin A: Broad examination plays exhibited the pivotal part of Vitamin A in thyroid wellbeing. This nutrient is fundamental for the union of thyroid chemicals and assumes a critical part in supporting the change of T4 (thyroxine) to the more dynamic

T3 (triiodothyronine) chemical. Contextual investigations have featured that a lack of Vitamin A can add to hypothyroidism.

Vitamin D: A lack of Vitamin D has been related to an expanded gamble of immune system thyroid issues. Studies propose that keeping up with ideal Vitamin D levels is significant for managing the resistant reaction and lessening irritation in the thyroid organ. Commonsense tips incorporate guaranteeing openness to daylight, dietary sources plentiful in Vitamin D or supplementation when important.

Vitamin B: The different B nutrients, especially B12 and B6, are fundamental for thyroid capability. They partake in the amalgamation and change of thyroid chemicals. Lack of these nutrients can prompt disturbances in thyroid chemical creation. Contextual analyses feature the relationship between B12 lack and hypothyroidism, stressing the significance of checking and enhancing when required.

Omega-3 Unsaturated fats: Omega-3 unsaturated fats, basically tracked down in greasy fish, flaxseeds, and pecans, assume a vital part in keeping up with hormonal equilibrium, including thyroid chemicals. Studies demonstrate that these unsaturated fats add to decreasing irritation, which is essential for forestalling immune system responses against the thyroid.

Reasonable tips incorporate integrating omega-3-rich food varieties into the eating routine or taking into account supplements. The Mediterranean eating routine, eminent for its accentuation on fish and plant-based fats, offers an outline for an eating routine helpful for thyroid wellbeing.

By getting it and carrying out these experiences into everyday nourishment, people can effectively add to the equilibrium of their thyroid chemicals, advancing in general prosperity and metabolic wellbeing. Ordinary checking of supplement levels, combined with an all-encompassing way to deal with nourishment, is vital to accomplishing and keeping up with thyroid concordance.

Part 6: DIETARY Procedures FOR GOITER The board.

Goiter, described by the broadening of the thyroid organ, frequently emerges from iodine inadequacy or other thyroid-related messes. This section investigates dietary procedures to oversee goitre, zeroing in on a goitre-accommodating eating routine improved with entire food sources.

Figuring out Goiter and Sustenance:

Before diving into dietary proposals, appreciating the connection between sustenance and goitre is critical. Iodine, a fundamental micronutrient, plays a crucial part in thyroid chemical combinations. An eating regimen lacking iodine can prompt thyroid brokenness, adding to goitre improvement. Furthermore, certain food sources, known as goitrogens, can slow down thyroid capability. Thus, a decent and cautiously organized diet is fundamental for goitre the board. Goiter-Accommodating Eating

Routine Arrangement:

Iodine-rich food sources: Incorporate iodine-rich food sources like ocean growth, iodized salt, fish, and dairy in your eating routine to guarantee a satisfactory iodine supply for thyroid capability.

<u>Calming Food varieties:</u> Settle food varieties with mitigating properties to moderate thyroid aggravation. Integrate natural products (berries, cherries), vegetables (salad greens, broccoli), and omega-3 unsaturated fats (greasy fish, flaxseeds).

<u>Limit Goitrogenic Food Sources:</u> While some goitrogenic food sources can be solid, control is critical. Limit admission of cruciferous vegetables (cabbage, broccoli), soy items, and certain organic products (peaches, strawberries).

Selenium Sources: Selenium is pivotal for thyroid wellbeing. Eat selenium-rich food sources like Brazil nuts, sunflower seeds, and lean meats.

<u>Entire Grains</u>: Accentuate entire grains like quinoa, earthy-coloured rice, and oats for supported energy and fibre, advancing general well-being.

<u>Recipes and Feast Thoughts</u>: Iodine-supporting serving of mixed greens:

Fixings: Ocean growth (nori or wakame), blended greens, cherry tomatoes, cucumber.

Dressing: Olive oil, lemon squeeze, a spot of iodized salt. Selenium-stuffed Pan fried food:

Fixings: Lean chicken/meat, broccoli, chime peppers, garlic.

Sauce: Soy sauce, ginger, and a sprinkle of squashed Brazil nuts.

Calming Smoothie:

Fixings: Berries, spinach, flaxseeds, Greek yogurt.

Discretionary: Add a teaspoon of honey for pleasantness.

Commonsense Tips:

Counsel a Nutritionist: Designer your eating routine arrangement in light of individual requirements. A nutritionist can give customized exhortations considering factors like age, orientation, and existing medical issues.

Hydration: Remain sufficiently hydrated, as water assumes a significant part in metabolic cycles, including thyroid capability.

<u>Ordinary Checking:</u> Intermittently evaluate thyroid capability through blood tests. Change your eating routine case by case in light of the outcomes and talk with medical care experts.

By taking on an all-encompassing way to deal with sustenance, consolidating iodine, overseeing goitrogenic food sources, and embracing mitigating decisions, people can add to goitre the executives. This part furnishes perusers with down-to-earth dietary techniques, building up the association between a supporting eating routine and thyroid well-being.

Part 7: Way of life CHANGES FOR GOITER Avoidance.

Goiter, a development of the thyroid organ, can be impacted by different way of life factors. Understanding and tending to these variables are vital for compelling avoidance. This dives into the complicated connection between way-of-life decisions and goitre improvement, giving contextual analyses and down-to-earth tips for perusers.

Way of Life Elements and Goiter

Iodine Admission: Low iodine levels are an essential driver of goitre. Contextual investigations from areas with iodine-lacking soils feature the predominance of goitre. Commonsense tips incorporate integrating iodine-rich food sources like kelp and iodized salt into the eating routine.

<u>Cruciferous Vegetables:</u> While these vegetables are by and large sound, over-the-top utilization can obstruct thyroid capability. The section investigates how adjusting cruciferous vegetable admission can relieve this gamble, referring to genuine models.

<u>Selenium Lack:</u> In regions with low selenium levels, goitre rates will quite often be higher. The part reveals insight into the significance of selenium and prompts on dietary sources and

supplementation where
fundamental.

The Job of Standard Activity

Metabolic Wellbeing: Exercise
helps with weight the board as
well as adds to metabolic
wellbeing. Contextual analyses
feature people who, through
standard active work, experienced
upgrades in thyroid capability and
a decreased gamble of goitre.

Safe Framework Tweak:
Exercise has invulnerable
balancing impacts, possibly
decreasing immune system-
related goitre. Reasonable tips
incorporate consolidating a blend
of high-impact and opposition

practices custom-made to individual wellness levels.
Stress The board for Goiter Avoidance

<u>Stress and Thyroid Capability:</u> Constant pressure can adversely affect thyroid well-being, adding to goitre improvement. The section examines the physiological components included and presents situations where stress decrease methods prompted upgrades.

<u>Mind-Body Practices:</u> Viable tips underscore the significance of psyche-body practices like reflection, yoga, and profound breathing activities. True models exhibit how people coordinated these practices into their ways of life.

Carrying out Way of Life Changes

Customized Approaches: Perceiving that every individual's way of life is interesting, the section urges perusers to take on customized approaches. Contextual investigations feature assorted procedures that people utilize to make a manageable way of life changes.

Coordinated effort with Medical services Experts: Underlining the cooperation among people and medical care experts, the part frames how clinical direction can improve the adequacy of the way of life intercessions. Useful hints incorporate standard well-being check-ups and observing thyroid capability.

By giving a thorough investigation of the way of life factors impacting goitre and offering proof-based tips, this part engages perusers to make proactive strides in forestalling and dealing with this thyroid condition.

Overseeing and forestalling goitre includes an exhaustive methodology that joins nourishing systems with clinical direction. It's pivotal to comprehend the fundamental reasons for goitre, which is frequently connected to iodine inadequacy yet can likewise be impacted by different factors like hereditary qualities and certain meds.

Part 8. Key Dietary Methodologies:

1. Iodine Admission:

Guarantee a sufficient admission of iodine, a fundamental part of thyroid chemical combination. Fish, iodized salt, dairy items, and kelp are great dietary sources. Be mindful not to consume unnecessary iodine, as this can likewise add to thyroid brokenness.

2. Selenium Supplementation:

Think about selenium supplementation, as it assumes a part in thyroid capability and can assist with diminishing irritation in the thyroid organ. Brazil nuts, fish, and sunflower seeds are normal wellsprings of selenium.

3. Cruciferous Vegetable Control:

Limit the admission of cruciferous vegetables (e.g., broccoli, cabbage) as they contain goitrogenic intensities that can impede thyroid capability. Cooking these vegetables can help lessen their goitrogenic impacts.

4. Adjusted Diet:

Keep an even eating routine wealthy in organic products, vegetables, lean proteins, and entire grains. This supports by and large wellbeing and gives fundamental supplements to thyroid capability.

<u>**Contextual analyses:**</u>
Case 1:

Sarah, determined to have iodine inadequacy goitre, effectively dealt with her condition by integrating iodine-rich food sources into her eating regimen and utilizing iodized salt. Ordinary checking guaranteed ideal iodine levels.

Case 2:

John, with an immune system thyroid confusion adding to his goitre, tracked down alleviation by remembering selenium-rich food varieties for his eating routine. Discussion with medical services proficiently aided in tailoring his nourishing arrangement to his particular requirements.

Useful Hints:

Normal Checking:

Intermittently check iodine levels through blood tests to guarantee ampleness without overabundance.

Screen thyroid capability through normal clinical check-ups.

Interview with Medical care Experts:

Look for direction from an endocrinologist or a medical care proficient gaining practical experience in thyroid issues.

Talk about individual dietary requirements and possible connections with drugs.

<u>Teach on Goiter Causes:</u>

Comprehend the different reasons for a goitre to customize healthful methodologies.
Teach the significance of resolving hidden issues for successful administration.

CONCLUSION

All in all, an all-encompassing way to deal with overseeing and forestalling goitre includes a cautious equilibrium between wholesome systems and clinical direction. Satisfactory iodine consumption, selenium supplementation, control of specific food varieties, and a reasonable eating regimen are key parts. It's significant to talk with medical care experts for customized exhortation and consistently screen thyroid capability. By joining wholesome mediations with clinical ability, people can enhance their way of

dealing with a goitre the board
and backing in general thyroid
wellbeing.